CORONA

What really kills us

BY

F.A THOMAS

TABLE OF CONTENT

4

INTRODUCTION

The trip to the doctor, the shopping for the week or a ride in the bus to work-everywhere we go nowadays we see the same picture i.e people with their faces and noses covered. Certainly these difficult times require these measures and along with protecting against the infection these measures provide other positive effects. But what are we protecting us from exactly ?

The invisible enemy

In the modern world where the traditional physical problems are no more there we fight a different kind of evil which is invisible, Cancer, viruses and bacteria, electrosmog and radioactivity are a few examples of these invisible modern enemies. An important role is played by the media, which steers the population to "their best" through targeted reporting. This authoritarian role is not always handled responsibly by the media. Only sensations and fear are processed and quickly spread by them. We can only form our own opinion based on what information is being feeded to us. if this information is manipulated and bundled, a collective thought process of our society emerges. The question arises if the media is leading the politicians or the politicians the media?

In this Covid -19 crisis the media has had a big hand . As discussed earlier Virus is one of the invisible enemies so is its infection. The only way people can understand the gravity of the situation is through mainstream media which is TV radio, newspaper etc.. They are the middle link of communication between the government and the public. The work of journalism was to provide as neutral as possible information along with rich perspectives including expression of error mistakes and criticism but this is hardly a reality nowadays. It must not be forgotten that the media has a power over our thought process and action.With the arrival of social media there has been a diverse opinion and algorithms find it difficult to ensure the diversity of the opinion. We make a perception on how we want it to be made and that is how we form our opinions.

The Mask- The new symbol of Unity ?

The corona measures have led us to behave in an uniform manner. Doesn't matter from where a person comes from, what his sexuality is, what his denomination or skin color is , the rules apply to everyone, that is distance and hygiene etiquettes. The group which benefits the most from these measures are elderly as they are the most vulnerable group as people have come together for protection of this group. However it is difficult to fight against some unconventional minded people. The same is right for other measures, which sometimes lead to disputes rather than unity.

Differences due to lack of differentiation

If the measures are justified they must be individually analysed for individual groups but there is hardly any differentiation present in decisions . Only the current inconsistent legislation makes a case-number-dependent, regional differentiation of the measures. Instead of the case-number haggling of the individual federal states, a uniform regulation according to risk groups is of far greater importance. The importance of an individual assessment of the measures is also made clear by Bodo de Vries, Chairman of DEVAP. "A differentiated view is necessary. Experts must be involved in this debate to know who and what challenges are at stake here. Over-sixty-year-old employees and 80-year-olds in inpatient care facilities cannot and must not be considered equally as a risk group." In this example, this requirement concerns only one social group, but it must also be applied to all others instead of collectively for hot spots according to case numbers. What is missing is a distinction of risk for different people. What are the disadvantages of exposing young and healthy while protecting the old and sick also needs to be discussed.

R-factor and total cases- key figures of the situation?

Collective fear is stoked to get everyone to isolate and vaccinate as well. But on what basis is this done? The number of cases is rising steadily, but what do they tell us? With an increasing number of tests, of course, the reported infection rate also increases. However it is not a clear indicator of the seriousness of the situation. If we take positive cases over total cases and get a percentage , it is a more realistic and practical approach and can lead to an objective actionable plan. Although this data is collected by RKI and is available on their website, mainstream media doesn't use it as an indicator. Instead they use the R factor which means the number of people infected by an infected individual. This approach is said to be not helpful. Moreover it's not generally understandable.

The incidence and death figures also show a high degree of uncertainty. "It naturally makes a difference weather a school class was infected or an old people's house; you just can't predict number of deaths by number of infected people" says Gérard Krause, head of epidemiology at the Helmholtz Centre for Infection Research in Braunschweig.

There is no case number of "pure" corona deaths. There are almost always pre-existing diseases present in a patient which add ons. This is also shown by a Germany-wide analysis by the AOK, that the percentage of people that had pre existing illnesses were higher in ventilated patients as compared to non ventilated patients after being affected by corona. Since the mortality rate is significantly higher in ventilated patients, a serious conclusion due to pre-existing conditions can be deduced.

A review of the number of deaths due to corona and related disease shows that a significant increase in the number of deaths occurs only in the age groups above 80 years. In young people, the number of deaths are comparatively lower.

Whether an objective assessment of the danger is at all desired by the political side remains questionable, since a political state of emergency can be hidden and justified behind the back of an unforeseeable pandemic.

Obedience at any price

How threatening is the virus really? Instead of just fighting with the virus alone and simply dealing with the consequences , we choose to remain together and follow the strict orders. For this, we accept massive restrictions on personal and economic freedoms, for a mortal danger that is only moderately justified. We enter into an obedience to protect "potential" casualties. How noble, how humane. But is it necessary? Or is life not life-threatening at all times?

Barbershops, schools, music clubs and sports clubs have to close, but professional sports continue. The sale of toys and electrical appliances is banned in supermarkets and some areas are even sealed off. Hair replacement is classified as relevant to the system, but washing the customer's hair before attaching a new hairpiece is considered a hairdressing service and therefore may not be performed as part of the permitted service. We obediently accept these and other decisions that were not individually analysed.

However, in the course of these strict measures, protests did not stop but increased. These protests are immediately dismissed as radical right-wing. Is it right-wing radical to question the necessity of measures that restrict freedom in particular? In a democracy, critical thinking must be allowed and its functioning absolutely needs critical thinking. Only then can arguments be reconsidered instead of being ignored and rules followed simply out of obedience.

Restrictions, bans and measures - they all influence our lives. But who are the real victims? Which sectors of our society are bearing the consequences of the pandemic and the changes it has brought? Ten of these groups will now be put under the microscope. Some aspects are widely known, but others would be somewhat fresh.

(1)CHRONICALLY PHYSICALLY ILL PEOPLE

Anyone who is ill must go to the doctor. A sentence that many people take for granted and should. This applies especially to people with chronic diseases. They need regular and more intensive medical care. But what if the grievance of doctors and nurses is repeatedly highlighted in the media? Shouldn't doctors be left to care for the "really sick"?

Misunderstood solidarity

Doctors' offices were already overcrowded before Corona, intensive care beds had just been removed by the private hospitals because they were too expensive for them to manage, and the shortage of doctors and nurses in Germany is well known and widespread. At this stage, a wave of disease is sweeping over us that is placing excessive demands on the entire health care system. Out of

misunderstood solidarity, there is a danger that the physically ill will no longer go to the doctor, or only in an emergency, in order to avoid having to use the doctor's manpower at the expense of the corona sick. In the worst case, even necessary doctor's appointments or operations are postponed despite complaints. The consequences are obvious. The state of illness of the person concerned can worsen considerably, consequential damage can occur or even lead to irreparable damage.

But is there a risk that one Corona patient will not be treated because of another? Is this fear justified? This question cannot be answered in a generalized way. Here, too, a differentiation must be made according to the disease and its severity. If we talk about chronic diseases that are treated by a general practitioner or specialist, there is probably no bottleneck here at present due to the rising corona numbers. However, the situation is different for patients who require regular hospital stays. In intensive care units in particular, some hospitals have already reached their upper limits. The situation is also worrying as far as ventilator capacity is concerned. The Süddeutsche Zeitung writes: "In Germany, ventilation capacity and the number of intensive care beds are being increased. But experts are uncertain whether this will be enough for all Covid 19 patients. Buying new ventilators is difficult at the moment - worldwide demand exceeds supply." So, at present, it cannot be determined that a decision will have to be made between two patients, as was the case in Italy in the spring of 2020. In addition, 1/3 of ventilated patients die, 1/3 suffer permanent damage and only 1/3 survive. This is also the reason why ventilation is now more cautious in the case of Covid-19 infection.

One thing is certain: anyone who needs help should see a doctor as soon as possible so as not to jeopardize their state of health and to receive care as quickly as possible. If this is neglected out of misunderstood consideration and the condition becomes even more critical, the cost of treatment can increase considerably and the initially well-intentioned restraint can lead to an even greater burden on the healthcare system

(2)GENERATION 80+

As already mentioned, the more severe courses of the disease mainly affect elderly people with pre-existing conditions. It is therefore only natural that the older generation is afraid of infection. The consequence of the fear is an increasing avoidance of contact with others.

A person, in the middle of life, goes to work, shopping, visiting friends and family, and is surrounded by people most of the day. Even during a pandemic, he can still maintain social contacts, at least to a limited extent, via social media and online meetings.

With retirement, however, a large proportion of contacts cease and are usually minimized to the circle of family and friends with increasing age. If a person isolates himself at this age, there are hardly any options. For fear of infection, any step outside the door is avoided and a visit is only granted to the closest family members. In the rarest cases, there is the possibility of communicating via the Internet, which leads to complete isolation. The result is an increase in the most common mental illness in old age: old-age depression.

Old people's home

If a person can no longer care for himself in old age and requires intensive care in everyday life, the nursing home is usually an inevitable decision for the relatives. Of course, there are also cases in which one or more family members take care of the relative, but this is not the rule and often hardly feasible.

Once there, the contact persons decrease drastically once again. The initially regular visits from the family with walks in the park eventually become short obligatory visits with cramped conversations, and the frequency also continues to decrease. The elderly are abandoned. Even if this is a view that no relative wants to confront, it cannot be dismissed out of hand. We don't take enough care of our elderly. This was already the case before Corona.

Finally, in the course of the Corona measures, the nursing homes were also temporarily closed.

Depending on the federal state, a resident may be visited at regular intervals by appointment only. In the case of a complete ban on visits, these people are left entirely alone. No visits. No treatments by therapists. No religious services. Depending on the state of health, it is not even possible for the person concerned to comprehend or assess the situation, which is why mental suffering is added to physical suffering.

The case numbers have also shown that nursing homes are a hotspot for the virus. Regular contact with nursing staff, who in turn also care for other patients, results in rapid spread in the event of infection. "According to the latest situation report from the Robert Koch Institute (RKI) on Monday evening, 55,931 people in nursing homes or homes for the elderly have been infected with Sars-CoV-2 so far

41,803 of whom are older than 60 years. Last Monday, the RKI reported 7447 fewer cases, when there were 48,484 total infected people, of whom 35,512 were older than 60. An increase of 15 percent." Focus reported on 24.12.2020.

The relatives' fear of the risk of infection therefore also minimizes the frequency of visits for this reason. For those affected, the few visits are a burden, but if one adds up the visitors who visit a nursing home every day, it quickly becomes clear that too many people nevertheless encounter each other directly or indirectly. At the current time, one person per resident is allowed to visit for one hour a day. With a facility of a hundred residents or more, that adds up to several thousand visitors each month. "We can't protect our residents sufficiently," says Heberger from the care company in this regard, admitting that it is accepted that more elderly people will become infected.

Often, the residents are also physically predisposed, which is why infection becomes a danger to life. So if the virus spreads throughout an entire facility, it places a massive burden on hospitals, as intensive care is often necessary.

Due to the incomplete reporting of the federal states, on the incidence of infection in nursing homes, a conclusive report can not yet be made. "The actual total number of affected homes is probably even significantly higher. Some states provided only incomplete figures, Berlin and Bavaria did not provide any information at all." says the Tagesschau in November 2020.

Rapid tests will now help limit the spread of the virus. Employees, visitors and residents are now to be regularly tested for Corona. The hurdle here, however, is bureaucracy and procurement. In order for the rapid tests to be reimbursed by the health insurance fund at a later date, the facility has to develop a testing concept, which has to be approved by the health department. This process leads to delays. According to a survey by the BIVA-Pflege Schutzbund on the use of rapid tests in Germany, less than five percent of the facilities that responded are already using them. In addition, there are supply bottlenecks because, unlike with protective materials, homes have to take care of procuring the tests themselves.

(3)PEOPLE WITH DISABILITIES

When one thinks of a disability, physical and mental limitations come to mind first and foremost. These, just like sick people, require increased care. Protective measures, such as the distance rule, cannot be observed between caregivers and patients. In addition to the increased risk of infection, it is hardly possible for people with mental disabilities to understand the new protective measures or to adhere to them at all.

Inclusion at risk

Above all, inclusion is at stake as a result of these measures. According to BAG WfbM, around 320,000 adults are currently in their member workshops. Almost 270,000 in the external work area. These are already included in the labor market. When the companies close, they now have to return to the workshops. In order to be able to apply for short-time working benefits, entrepreneurs have to cut outside jobs. Those who suffer are the disabled people, for whom there are no compensation payments. In terms of inclusion, this is an enormous step backwards. The workshops are then the only safety net.

However, some of these facilities will also be closed and those affected in this case will be unemployed. The closure of the workshops was justified by the containment of the pandemic. In this case, those affected lose their jobs and social contacts with like-minded people. According to the Federal Employment Agency, this affected about thirteen percent more in November than in the previous year of the same month. It is difficult for these people to find their way back into the labor market.

In the case of an intellectual disability, it is difficult for those affected to understand what is happening and for what reasons measures are being taken. "Many people with disabilities belong to the vulnerable group and have a right to understandable information," said Jürgen Dusel, Federal Disability Commissioner.

But let's think ahead - disabilities cover a much broader spectrum.

Do you get what i am saying ?

A deaf person communicates through sign language, that is, through signs that are performed with the hands. Right? Not only! Sign language is a visual, natural language with its own grammar. It is a pictorial and vivid language that combines signs, facial expressions, gestures, mouth images and body language and is the only way to communicate thoughts, feelings, complicated issues and topics. To communicate, you need eye contact from the other person. This way, the person knows that he or she is being addressed and can follow the conversation.

If you watch a broadcast on TV with a sign language interpreter, you can see that she doesn't just move her hands. She communicates with her entire upper body. The facial expressions, the gestures and the posture - all these things are part of the expression and understanding of a deaf person.

If two deaf people want to talk to each other in public and have to wear a mask, half of the information contained in the mask is lost and communication is considerably disturbed.

This barrier begins in communication with others of this language and extends into everyday life with hearing people. How can a deaf person communicate with hearing people if they do not know sign language? At this point, the deaf person reads from the lips of the other person. The reproduction is then done by sounds that imitate a spoken language and can be understood by hearing people. If the reading of the lips and facial expressions is omitted due to the wearing of a mask, communication is completely impossible. Even if the interlocutor tries to communicate through gestures, he or she is often misunderstood, creating an even greater barrier. Shopping, a visit to the office or doctor, the bus ride to work - these are all situations in which communication is now no longer possible.

Do you feel what i am saying?

Another form of disability is blindness. In this case, the person is dependent on the help of those who guide him. Proximity is therefore indispensable in this situation, when a blind person wants to find his way without the familiarity of the surroundings.

It is extremely remarkable what our fellow human beings with disabilities are capable of. Is it lip reading or orientation by means of hearing, or with the help of a cane for the blind. If these possibilities are taken away from them, they are more helpless than ever.

In the Corona consultation process of the German Association for Rehabilitation (DvfR), with the support of the Federal Ministry of Labor and Social Affairs (BMAS), the experienced effects of the Corona pandemic on people with disabilities are currently being examined from various perspectives. People with disabilities, relatives, rehabilitation facilities, umbrella organizations, service and cost providers, and representatives of civil society were surveyed. Participation in the survey was possible until December 13, 2020. An evaluation will not take place until next year, but this can provide a basis for further political action with a connection to reality and contribute to the inclusion of our society.

(4) MENTALLY ILL PEOPLE

It is not only people with physical limitations who are affected by the current situation. For those who already suffer from depression, anxiety disorders or other diseases of the soul, it also has a strong impact. The latest survey by the University of Basel, which examines the psychological burden of the second Covid 19 wave, found that the number of people with severe depressive symptoms has doubled from 9% to 18%. The April and November 2020 values were compared. If one adds the value of 3%, which was determined before the pandemic, the value even increased sixfold. In addition, young people, who suffered financial losses in the course of the pandemic, are particularly affected.

The soul carousel

Often depressed people withdraw into themselves, avoid all social contact, as well as physical activities. Even the daily work routine is no longer manageable for some. This situation is exacerbated by the loss of contact opportunities. However, a social environment of friends and family is extremely important for mentally ill people, as they need the support, understanding and also the motivation of others.

The consequence here is also a deterioration of the state of health. Negative thoughts circle more and more like a merry-go-round. You move around, but you still don't make any progress. The more the depression intensifies, the less it is possible for those affected to get out of this mood on their own.

In order to give each other support and stability, group therapy is used in psychosomatic clinics in particular, but also in outpatient practices. Conflict situations, fears, hurdles in everyday life and the clinical picture itself are discussed, but joint activities are also planned. In the sheltered atmosphere of people who can understand one's own situation, thought processes and fears. However, since these are hardly feasible, this support is no longer needed.

Without a job, without regular meetings with other affected persons and without the help of friends, not only the social contacts are missing, but also the occupations. Again the merry-go-round turns. Again, negative thoughts and feelings are circling.

For mentally healthy people, the Corona pandemic is a real ordeal. Some employees are losing their jobs, others are working from home, and still others have been put on short-time work for an indefinite period. A situation that is unquestionably stressful.

Mutual support- but with corona restrictions

"We should now pay attention to our fellow human beings who may suffer from loneliness and social isolation in the coming weeks. How is your neighbor, maybe offer support, e.g. [...] Do you need help with the shopping? " is the advice of HU expert Prof. Dr. Ulrike Lüken. Those who are acutely affected can still seek help promptly. Lüken cites examples such as the telephone counselling service, the crisis service, the child and youth telephone, and online therapies. These are Corona-compliant and more quickly accessible than appointments with therapists and psychiatrists. Nevertheless, there is no substitute for personal contact for people with mental health problems with a doctor or therapist.

(5) YOUNG PEOPLE

How does the pandemic affect the younger generation, who have no physical ailments or financial problems? They, too, are among the Corona victims.

The development phases

The developmental stages of a young child span five levels. Sensory development, motor development, social development, emotional development and cognitive development. Let's take a brief look at each of them separately.

Sensory integration refers to the perceptual areas of tasting, hearing, seeing, feeling and spatial orientation. All these impressions have to be processed to get an impression of the environment. However, they are also necessary for the development of other abilities, such as speech.

The area of movement processes are assigned to motor skills. It includes drinking, eating (chewing), swallowing, grasping, speaking, walking and more. Especially the oral motor skills are significant for speech and voice development.

Social development means the ability to build relationships with other people. From the very beginning, children learn to build trusting relationships with caregivers who serve as role models in both behavior and communication.

The ability to perceive and express different feelings is called emotional competence, which must be learned in childhood. Emotional and social development are closely interwoven and thus overlap. The German Federal Association for Speech Therapy says: "A child who acquires a trusting relationship and strong attachment to his caregivers learns early positive feelings, such as interest, joy, surprise, while a child with little attachment learns primarily feelings such as shame, fear, contempt or guilt. For the child's language development, positive emotional development is important as an expression of a strong attachment, so that the child accepts the parents as communication partners and learns from them.

The intellectual ability "[...] to recognize and classify objects, situations, people, including oneself, is called cognitive development.

Some functions of cognitive development are abstract thinking such as problem solving,language, memory, action planning or perceptual ability." (Deutscher Bundesverband für Logopädie e.V.)

Conclusion

It is therefore clear that each individual area affects the further development of a child into adulthood. If one building block is now removed, all the others can still hold the structure, but it ultimately becomes unstable. In terms of the Covid 19 pandemic, these building blocks are social bonding with other children and educators, which can no longer be fully developed. Another building block is the habit of wanting to explore, feel, and put everything in the mouth. As described above, this is indispensable for motor development, but should be avoided at all costs due to the current risk of infection. The result is an unstable structure of only partially learned skills, which is reflected in language deficits, attachment difficulties, lack of empathy and other emotional states as well as other abnormalities.

Our school children

Young children are already among the big victims. Kindergartens were closed for months or were only open for emergency care. Social contact with peers and friends was limited or nonexistent for weeks. Future elementary school students were unable to say goodbye to their teachers in the usual way after kindergarten ended. For kindergarten children, the transition to school time is special. Normally, future students can get to know their future schools and teachers in advance, and conversely, many teachers can get to know their future students. This year, all of this has only been possible to a limited extent or has even been eliminated.

Starting school is usually celebrated in a big way in Germany. It means a change from being a child to a student. This new situation is a joyful event, but it is also a challenge for those who are still young. They first have to find their way in the new world and learn their place in the system. This is once again interrupted by the renewed closure of the schools. Having just arrived, students and teachers once again become estranged. Friendships that were in the process of forming cannot deepen, as they cannot be deepened in the private sphere either due to the Corona regulations.

Another topic is distance learning. Learning letters and numbers and discovering, marveling at and experiencing many "aha" effects together can only be felt and experienced in a group setting. It needs exchange and reflection with peers, instead of only with annoyed parents at home.

Many skills can only be learned in a group. Above all, the ability to deal with conflict is particularly developed during the school years. Arguments with classmates and discussions with teachers are just as much a part of development as group work. Disputes with classmates are important for social competence, as this is where argumentation skills, assertiveness and empathy are trained. In the relationship between student and teacher, critical faculties and the ability to subordinate oneself are also acquired. Group work also develops social skills. They learn to work in a team and to adapt to each other. They also learn to accept other points of view and to be open to them. It is about dealing with the opinions of others and finding common solutions in a team to achieve goals. Many of these opportunities are now severely limited or eliminated altogether.

Conclusion

The social learning effect, in terms of teamwork, critical thinking and argumentation skills, is taken away from our school children. Many of these learning processes cannot be fully developed and learned, which becomes noticeable in later everyday work. They may not be able to withstand confrontations with colleagues and the boss, which results in diminished self-confidence. It may be difficult to work on tasks in a structured manner, and instead of working as a team, everyone does their own thing. Whether or not we'll see a generation of disorganized lone wolves, to put it bluntly, depends on the course and long-term consequences of the pandemic and will only become clear in the next few years.

Puberty

What's the first thing that comes to an adult's mind when they think of a pubescent child? Stubbornness, pushing boundaries, intense friendships, interest in the opposite sex, and intensive use of the Internet, game consoles, and smartphones. As dating, as well as meeting friends, becomes severely limited, the range of interests of adolescents continues to shift toward gaming and Internet addiction. The numbers of addicted users also rose steadily in previous years, but quarantine or simply staying in one's own home more often encourages technology dependent behavior in all age groups.

The health insurer DAK presented a study on this, which revealed that the usage time of children and adolescents between ten and seventeen years, during the contact restriction, increased from 79 to 139 minutes, i.e. by 75 percent. The figures were compared from September 2019 and May 2020, the peak of the first Corona wave. Moreover, this increase refers only to online gaming. Social media use increased from just under two hours to over three hours. Is this really what we want our kids to learn?

Only on cell phones?

During the lockdown, the cell phone was and still is the only way for many young people to communicate with their circle of friends. According to Dr. Gabriele Komesker, head of the child protection outpatient clinic at the Protestant Hospital in Düsseldorf, contacts with the peer group are the most important and cannot be replaced. "Teenagers want to hang out with each other, get close. That was taken away from them from one moment to the next and has certainly increased the feeling of loneliness in many," says Komesker. Above all, if children and adolescents already had a hard time making friends before the pandemic, they are particularly at risk of loneliness.

Dr. Kemesker is also critical of the increasing virtual contacts and says: "Social media were certainly a help in times of limited contacts, but just not for everyone. In addition, it must always be considered whether the time spent in front of the screens was controlled and limited or not. The longer the exclusively virtual contact lasts and the more the young people seem to be absorbed in it, the higher the probability of addiction."

The day-night rhythm of many young people is also disrupted by going to bed much later and sleeping in too late. This can make it all the more difficult to get back into a regular routine.

Of particular concern is the increasing risk of cyberbullying and abuse of minors. Often, there is no control over their interaction and the content they consume, which is why they can move around the web without restriction. Our children and young people are freely exposed to chats with complete strangers as well as hostility from others. Parents in particular should be aware of which platforms their children are using so that they can intervene in good time.

Conclusion

In adolescence, corona determinations have a particularly strong effect on a sharp increase in Internet and computer game use. This in turn increases the risk of depression, according to the study by health insurer DAK. Other consequences include reduced performance, impaired family life and friendships, neglect of hobbies, and aggression and irritability. For these reasons, the healthcare system is increasingly focusing on early detection and prevention.

(6)PARTNERSHIP

Spending more time than usual with your loved ones, especially your partner, can cause tension. But how much time is too much of a good thing?

The fiction between partners

Couples spend much more time together during the pandemic and are now forced to adjust and deal with each other and their wishes. This can lead to frustration and disappointment. Those annoying habits that were otherwise endearing as long as you only had to put up with them at closing time now become the trigger for arguments and underlying anger. The pile of laundry in the corner of the living room, which could otherwise be dismissed with a shake of the head, can now lead to heated arguments.

Even old problems that have been lying dormant beneath the surface now come to light and are amplified as if with a magnifying glass. If conflicts arise due to the constant closeness, it is also difficult to avoid each other. Leisure activities and even visits to friends, to whom one could lament one's suffering and find support, now fall away. The anger continues to accumulate, which can lead to serious problems in the partnership, far beyond the lockdown.

Conflicts should therefore be resolved as quickly as possible so as not to jeopardize the relationship. In addition, measures can be taken to lower one's own stress level so as not to go to the limit again the next time a dispute arises.

Even if the problems are not in the partnership itself, they affect it. People who feel unwell, have financial anxieties, experience professional stress or are lonely also show this. Either through irritability, sadness and hopelessness or emotional withdrawal. In the latter case, open conflict does not occur, but the withdrawal distances both partners from each other when they no longer communicate with the other.

However, there is also a positive aspect. Both can use the time together to bring common rituals back into the relationship. For example, eating together, planning new activities after the lockdown, or redecorating your home can help you get through this time harmoniously, creatively, and productively. However, your own free space is also particularly important. Phone calls with friends, your own hobbies within the bounds of what is feasible, and your own time on a walk create time to escape the permanent couple time.

A new love is like a new life

That's how Jürgen Marcus sang it in his song from 1972. But how do you meet a new love in the days of Corona? Sure, online dating existed long before Corona, but even there, real meetings happen sooner or later. Besides, getting to know each other via online platforms is not a desirable alternative for everyone.

Once you have overcome the first hurdle of online dating and met a potential partner, you usually meet for a coffee, later for a romantic meal, and at some point privately in your own apartment. So far so good. But now things get serious.

Any proximity is a risk factor, even more so when tenderness is exchanged. Coronaviruses are transmitted by droplet infection, which is unavoidable during sex. It is also impossible to determine whether a person is contagious, because the disease sometimes runs without symptoms. In this way, the virus can spread unnoticed. The fear of this possibility thus complicates sexual life and dating in general.

(7) VICTIMS OF DOMESTIC VIOLENCE

The restrictions on contact put a strain on social life within the family. The fact that this can lead to frequent conflicts was described in the previous chapter. Work, household chores, childcare and financial fears create a multiple burden. Often, problems can be discussed and the smoke clears. But what if it doesn't? What if fear and anger rise to the point of physical or psychological violence?

Does corona lead to higher levels of violence?

"We still do not have any reliable figures for Germany on the extent to which the measures to combat the Corona virus have led to more domestic violence. During the first lockdown, women sought less help, partly out of fear of becoming infected in the women's shelter," says Johanna Thie, an expert at Diaokonie Deutschland.

Even if there are figures on domestic violence in the coming weeks or months, they will not be very meaningful. Only cases that are reported can be included in the statistics. However, if the victim does not dare to accept help for fear of infecting himself or others, these cases can neither be investigated nor the victims helped.

In this case, education is important. Affected persons must have the certainty that they can get help without posing a risk to themselves or others. "Our women's shelters and counseling centers are well prepared for the first lockdown: Hygiene plans have been drawn up, alternative quarters have been rented and much more. In order to implement the contact ban, face-to-face counseling had to be partially switched to telephone or online counseling" This was said about the assistance provided by the Diakonie.

But the attention of neighbors, relatives and friends is also very important. Of course, not every argument leads to domestic violence, but observers should act if they have reasonable suspicion. For example, they could first make contact by telephone. If the situation threatens to escalate, however, help from the police, counseling centers and women's shelters should always be called in.

Violence in children

If children are involved in domestic violence, the situation is much more precarious. The Tagesspiegel speaks of increasing indications of violence against children and young people. Here, too, the number of unreported cases is high, since children are not able to take responsibility for themselves and seek help.

DJI researchers, who evaluated scientific articles, position papers of professional associations and first results of empirical studies, came to the following conclusion: "The continuous personal contact between child protection professionals and families, which is particularly affected by infection control, is difficult to replace" (Report from Child Protection Lower Saxony in October 2020).

The search for creative solutions

Personal contact cannot be replaced by the media. In order to be able to help affected adults and children despite the restrictions on contact, the necessary technology must be made available in the counseling centers. " The establishment of digital counseling formats is not possible now. They are currently being tested and which would support young people and families in the long term, even in times of social distancing." Birgit Jentsch and Brigitte Schnock wrote this in an article in the September issue of the journal Child Abuse and Neglect. What is still doable today is contribution to simplifying and expanding counseling channels and reducing the number of unreported cases in the future.

(8) HOBBY AND FITNESS- CONSEQUENCES OF LACK OF EXERCISE

During the pandemic, gyms, sports fields, clubs and recreational facilities have closed. As a result, hobbies and sports can no longer take place as they used to. This has consequences for the body, the psyche and the economy.

Rising healthcare costs

"With the accompanying increase in inactivity, corresponding negative consequences for health and additional health care costs of around 1.8 billion euros are to be expected," according to the DIFG (Deutscher Industrieverband für Fitness und Gesundheit e.V.). But what are the consequences of a lack of inactivity for each individual?

Muscle loss

Our body builds muscles as soon as they are regularly and progressively stressed. However, muscles are a luxury good for the body, which it breaks down again during inactivity. So if the body is no longer challenged in the form and intensity, the hard-earned muscle mass begins to break down.

Increased risk of stroke

A large-scale study from the USA concluded that physical inactivity is almost as harmful as smoking. The study examined risk factors for cardiovascular disease and stroke in different ethnic groups. The risk of stroke was said to be increased by 65% with physical inactivity.

Tension

If muscles are no longer loaded, the muscles of the spine and the entire musculoskeletal system, which are responsible for the stability of our joints, also atrophy. This results in incorrect posture and strain. These are particularly evident when slouching on sofas and in beds in unnatural postures while consuming multimedia. This is accompanied by an increased risk of injury, as well as tension-related head, back and neck pain. In the worst case, it can even lead to a slipped disc.

Digestive complaints

In order for our digestion to run smoothly, a balanced diet and regular exercise are necessary. Exercise ensures good blood circulation in our organs. If the day is spent almost exclusively sitting, the organs become compressed. As a result, they can no longer develop freely, which can lead to digestive problems.

Obesity and Diabetes

Lack of exercise results in reduced calorie consumption. The metabolism slows down and the energy requirement decreases. If the amount of food consumed remains the same, there is an imbalance between calorie intake and consumption. This means that more calories are consumed than the body needs. This in turn leads to weight gain, resulting in obesity, which is the most common cause of diabetes mellitus. Adjusting eating behavior to physical exertion is one possibility. However, to maintain energy needs, regular exercise should be incorporated into everyday life. A walk after lunch and at the end of the day, as well as regular exercise, prevents a shock on the scales and secondary diseases.

Stress

Stress hormones are released in the body when it is exposed to stress. This leads to a brief increase in performance. However, these stress hormones must be reduced again, otherwise the permanent stress will lead to further physical consequences. The new situation causes more stress than we already have to cope with in everyday life. This should be reduced by exercise and sports. It is the valve that lets our stress level sink and gives us new strength for the next day. If this does not happen, there will be consequential damage caused by stress.

Osteoarthritis and osteoporosis

Lack of exercise can lead to joint wear and tear (osteoarthritis), as the cartilage in our joints suffers from the lack of movement and metabolic products can no longer be removed. Moderate stress through sports and general exercise in everyday life counteracts osteoarthritis.

Osteoporosis leads to a decrease in bone density and is therefore also referred to as bone loss. This makes the skeleton more susceptible to bone fractures. The disease can be counteracted by exercise, since bone substance builds up where there is a strain on the muscles.

Many people want to exercise and are looking for alternatives. Physical exercise is important for the psyche and the body, especially in the pandemic, to reduce stress and provide variety in everyday life. It is therefore not surprising that the sale of sports equipment for home use has increased sharply.

Fitness equipment as a box office hit

"For large equipment such as ergometers, the increase in April was about 80 percent. Most popular were classics such as weights with barbells and dumbbells but also fascia rollers, yoga mats or jump ropes. Sales of these smaller utensils rose by 300 percent." says an article at ntv.

Fitness boom in the living room

Training plans are structured and the nutrition plan is precisely coordinated. If the training in the gym is omitted, it comes to a disbalance and muscle loss. To counteract this, ambitious athletes and fitness trainers in particular rely on home workouts. Often, even online training sessions are offered free of charge by the gym, in order to be able to offer their customers something even during the closure.

(9)THE WORKPLACE

As already mentioned, many employees struggle with financial shortages due to short-time work or even the loss of their jobs. The social aspect of not being able to talk to colleagues also contributes to far-reaching consequences.

Working time is lifetime

Work is not only a way to earn money, it is also the place where we spend half of our day. If this space is limited by online meetings instead of face-to-face interaction, the quality of life decreases as well. Of course, everyone is happy to be able to work in a home office for a few days, but when one's own home becomes a permanent workplace, the social aspects that a workday in the office would bring are eliminated. The casual conversation at the coffee machine, the convivial lunch break with colleagues or the brief exchange over a smoke - all these otherwise unnoticed everyday relationships are then gone. Colleagues and business partners can now only be greeted at online meetings. However, these are no substitute for a relaxed conversational atmosphere. Home offices also change family life. Fixed working hours and childcare plays a role in working hours.

Information loss

Since, as already mentioned, direct exchange is eliminated and only takes place online, conversations are reduced to a necessary minimum. The work-related topics that are necessary to perform the work are still discussed, but any personal and private components are lost. Information is bundled in such a way that a comprehensive picture of issues can only be presented to a very limited extent. So you know when and how to do what work, but the casual conversation with colleagues about their experiences, views and suggestions is eliminated. As a result, much of the potential and innovation falls by the wayside.

Gestures and facial expressions can also not be fully reproduced by the screen, on which the conversation partner is only partially visible, which can distort a comprehensive exchange of information. Likewise, poor sound and image reproduction can become an obstacle in the home office.

Get out of the comfort zone

Usually, stepping out of your comfort zone is an opportunity to gain further knowledge and skills. However, if a home office worker is left to deal with the technical challenges on his or her own, it can become overwhelming. Especially for older people who aren't as tech-savvy as their younger colleagues, the sudden transition adds stress. Even setting up the computer for an online meeting can lead to helplessness and anger.

New tasks are usually introduced through training. This gives the employee time to get to grips with what is new and to adjust to the situation. In a lockdown, however, this introduction cannot take place. In some cases, employees are directly instructed to go to the home office and have to master the situation on their own.

Companies in which the home office was already part of everyday life before the Corona crisis, on the other hand, are well prepared and therefore have fewer teething problems. If the new workplace arrangement proves successful, however, there may be an opportunity for an individual and flexible working time model in the future. However, this will never be able to replace a personal workplace.

Work with customers

In businesses with customer contact, such as medical practices, the interplay between control and communication is particularly important. Although everyone is informed about the necessary hygiene measures in the media, conflicts between staff and customers still occur time and again. Employees are instructed to enforce and control compliance with their customers' measures, as well as to fulfill all requirements themselves. This undoubtedly means more work and stress. Customers who forget to abide by these rules or simply refuse to accept them add to the burden. Reminding a customer to put on a mask or disinfect his or her hands may still be justifiable, but a policy discussion about the usefulness of such regulations, which in the worst case could lead to the customer being ejected, can make everyday work more difficult. Nevertheless, employees with constant customer contact are exposed to such situations again and again. Balancing courteous customer service with strict authority is an art that tests employees, especially now. However, this must not turn out in such a way that the service provider mutates into the executive of Corona regulations.

(10) THE ECONOMY

Rising unemployment figures, many employees on short-time work, a slump in sales and increasing sick leave are not only a burden on employees, but also on companies and the economy.

Out of the black?

If our country has been in the black recently, the situation is now more strained. High costs due to unemployment figures and short-time working allowances, a healthcare system in full swing and a lack of taxes due to a slump in sales are just a few examples that are weighing on our country's bank account. "Instead of the originally planned waiver of any new loans as part of the debt brake, the 16 state parliaments have approved a possible new debt of up to 128 billion euros for 2020 alone, with several states wanting to stretch the borrowing over several years," it says in the Frankfurter Allgemeine of Dec. 20, 2020. The front-runner, it says, is Bavaria, which has claimed almost a third of the sum approved by the state parliaments with 40 billion euros in new debt. However, the states want to spread the amount of debt they have taken on over several years.

In addition to the state treasury, many companies in a wide variety of industries are short of cash. Let's take a closer look at a few of them.

The food industry

As part of the cross-national measures to limit the spread of the virus, the hospitality industry has been closed. In the wake of the loss of sales, some businesses have already had to close. The financial burden was too high. Those who can, are responding flexibly to the new situation. Many restaurants offer pick-up and delivery services to keep the store running, as the saying goes. But the economic situation is not pretty even when such creative solutions are found.

The tourism industry

Many countries are on the list with global travel warning. As a result, the tourism industry has been severely affected by the Corona pandemic, such as tour operators, the hotel industry, and the aviation and shipping industries. Especially aviation is doubly punished, as they have to comply with restrictions on passenger and, moreover, cargo traffic.

Exhibition and event industry

Gatherings of people are prohibited, which particularly affects the event industry. Events such as concerts, trade fairs and opera performances have been canceled. This affects the companies, but also in particular the freelance performers and artists, who can hardly hope for compensation.

The regional trade

While online retailing, and here especially Amazon, is booming and additionally cashing in on the sales figures of regional stores, many other companies are coming under severe pressure. Sales are completely lost due to the closures, which not all entrepreneurs can afford over a longer period of time. Many businesses suffered particularly in the past Christmas season, in which they had generated a large proportion of their sales (over 30%) on just a few days in previous years. It was precisely this revenue that was lost due to store closures at Christmas time.

Companies in the service sector

Hair salons, nail salons, pedicures and beauty salons - they all had to close their doors. Small businesses and sole proprietorships, which have been deprived of their livelihood, have been hit particularly hard. But even larger businesses, such as physiotherapy practices, are struggling with the high drops in sales.

The threat to the existence of companies also has far-reaching consequences for their employees. Unemployment and the associated psychological consequences characterize the year.

Unemployment

The corona-related increase in unemployment alone shows the impact of the economic situation. Spring usually sees a seasonal drop in unemployment. Nevertheless, according to the Labor Agency, the number increased by 20.5% between March and May 2020. Exact figures reflecting corona-related unemployment are not currently available. A simplified method that compares the figures with the previous year alone results in an increase in the unemployment rate of 1.3 percentage points.

In the event of a job loss, the first port of call is usually the employment agency. However, the agency is regularly closed and only admits people with an appointment. On the one hand, unemployment registration is done online, which becomes a hurdle for many of those affected. On the other hand, direct contact with the counselor is no longer necessary. If an employee wants to quit, for example, because of psychological stress at work, he will not receive timely personal counseling through the employment agency. If he quits anyway in his distress, unemployment benefits are blocked for up to twelve weeks. The person in question cannot present his reasons in person and find joint solutions with the counselor. Instead, he is left to his own devices in this situation and can only describe his situation to a complete stranger by e-mail or on the phone. This is certainly only one example of many possible scenarios in which employees who are affected by unemployment or the threat of it need personal and quick help, but do not receive it.

Resumé

As can be seen from the discussions, a pandemic, the consequences of which will probably not be known conclusively for years to come, is a heavy burden for every individual, as well as for companies and the economy. The education and development of children and young people is at risk, the rapidly increasing number of cases spreads fear and puts the healthcare system to a severe test. Psychological stress, which can lead to problems in partnerships and even domestic violence, are also effects of this crisis. The decisive factor is how we deal with it and what solutions we find. Some things are in our own hands.

Critical expression of opinion must be followed

Many people now decide to express their anger publicly. Critical statements testify to the desire for a self-determined life and the ability to critically question circumstances. These voices must be allowed, instead of dismissing them as right-wing extremists or conspiracy theorists - which seems to be the same thing. A good example of how to respond to legitimate protests is the city of Chemnitz. After protests against the influx of immigrants became loud, fears and anger were also expressed in racist terms. The city nevertheless took action and held regular citizens' meetings. At each table sat a politician who talked to citizens on a particular topic. People of all ages and social classes came to the meeting.

Whether the suggestions made a difference is not clear, but it was shown that a government can listen if it wants to. Examples like this certainly exist in other cities. This approach can be expanded and gives people the feeling that they are being taken seriously instead of having decisions imposed on them.

Recognizing opportunities where others see only limitations.

The catering industry shows the way; it creates alternative options. If no guests can be admitted, the food can be delivered or picked up. There are certainly no quick fixes for every industry, but now is the time to rethink and see opportunities. In the meantime, platforms are emerging that support regional trade. Retailers can offer their goods and services on them. Often, smaller stores cannot compete with the prices of wholesalers who offer their products on large marketplaces. However, those who value supporting their region can shop regionally even now online. Companies are forced to follow the change that already exists and explore new avenues. This benefits the customers.

Teaching at schools is now also becoming increasingly digitized. This has its downsides, but the widespread provision of technical aids for schools and students is helping children learn to use media efficiently and responsibly.

The situation is similar in companies whose employees work in a home office. It may be hard to get started, but digitization and with it the implementation of more flexible working time models is being driven forward. Just a year ago, home office days were hard to imagine for many companies. Now, however, there is an opportunity to test, elaborate and improve the home office model. Some companies have even said they have had good experiences with it and plan to continue giving their employees this option even after the pandemic. This has advantages for both sides. For example, the employee doesn't have to take a vacation just because his car won't start in the morning, or can complete tasks for which he needs rest and concentration at home. The employer, on the other hand, can calculate more cost-efficiently. For example, he can provide free workstations that employees can use on a rotating basis. Here, too, opportunities and solutions must be sought.

After the normal -Back to normal

The federal government intends to vaccinate at least 60% of the population to achieve herd protection. Once this is completed, the measures of contact restrictions should also be obsolete. Social and physical contact, i.e. celebrating together, hugging, kissing, creating new encounters - all this is essential for a fulfilled life. So it is necessary to make up for what has been missed. The fellowship of those we love is what makes our lives worth living. And that's what we're taking back.

Sozial.de - The news portal Online article from 03.08.2020

German radio

AOK Federal Association GbR Press release 29.07.2020

German Health Portal Online article from 15.12.2020 Online article from 17.12.2020

German Federal Association for Speech Therapy e.V.
South German Newspaper
German Industry Association for Fitness and Health e.V.
n-tv Nachrichtenvernsehen GmbH

Online article from 09.05.2020
- Diakonie Germany

Online article from 17.12.2020
- Internet portal child protection in Lower Saxony

Project of the Lower Saxony Ministry for Social Affairs, Health and Equality to intensify child protection in Lower Saxony

Online article from 29.10.2020

- Office Fitness
Online article: 12 consequences of lack of fitness

- Hans Böckler Foundation

Online article: Labor Market in Transition: Corona Consequences: Rise in Unemployment
- Federal Statistical Office

Economic impact - statistics related to Covid-19.

- **Frankfurter Allgemeine Zeitung GmbH** Online article from 20.12.2020

-   **Daytime news**
-   Federal working group

Workshops for disabled people e.V. Online article from 07.08.2020

- **North Rhine Medical Association** Online article from 23.10.2020 - Lokalkompass

FUNKE NRW Wochenblatt GmbH Online article from 11.11.2020

- **FinCompare GmbH**
    Online article from 23.0